Sugar Detox

Sugar Detox Program: Beat Sugar Craving, Lose Weight & Feel Less!

By: Samantha Michaels

Table of Contents

Introduction 5

Chapter 1: Preliminaries and Self-Assessment 7

    Types of Sugar 7

        Sucrose 7

        Fructose 8

        Glucose 8

        Lactose 9

        Galactose 9

        Other Sugars 9

    Moderation 9

    Sugar Addiction Quizzes 10

        Quiz 1: Assessment for Type 1 Sugar Addiction 10

        Quiz 3: Assessment for Type 3 Sugar Addiction 15

        Quiz 4: Assessment for Type 4 Sugar Addiction 17

Chapter 2 Sugar Addiction 22

    What is Sugar Addiction? 22

    Types of Sugar Addiction 23

        Type 1 23

        Type 2 24

- Type 3 24
- Type 4 24
- There is Hope for the Sugar Addicts 25
- Chapter 3 Sugar Detox 26
  - What Is Sugar Detox? 26
  - An Overview of Sugar Detox 27
- Chapter 4 Why Sugar Detox 29
  - Medical or Therapeutic Benefits 29
  - Physical Benefits 30
  - Emotional and Mental Benefits 30
- Chapter 5 Why Sugar is Dangerous for Weight Loss 31
- Chapter 6 Who will Benefit from Sugar Detox? 33
- Chapter 7 Natural Sugar Alternatives 34
  - The Artificial Sweetener Scare: How They Work 34
  - The Best Natural Sweeteners 34
    - Stevia 34
    - Xylitol 36
    - Coconut Palm Sugar 36
- Chapter 8 The Sugar Detox Plan in a Nutshell: What to Eat, Not to Eat and How to Eat 38
  - What to Eat and Drink 38
  - What to Not to Eat and Drink 40

Dos 42

How to Eat 43

Chapter 9 15-Day Meal Plan for Sugar Detox 44

Chapter 10 Dermal Detox 54

Channels of Detoxification 54

The Skin's Role in the Detox Process 55

Chapter 11 The Sugar-Exercise Connection 57

Recommended Exercise for Sugar Detox 57

Benefits of Exercise in Sugar Detox 57

The Sugar-Exercise Connection 58

Chapter 12 Maintenance Plan 59

Chapter 13 How to Dine Out with Sugar Detox Diet 60

Chapter 14 Some Sugar Detox Recipes 62

Introduction

The world is under siege by the onslaught of diabetes, which the World Health Organization now considers as a global epidemic. There are 347 million people afflicted with diabetes and 9 out of every 10 of all cases are Type II diabetes, largely as a consequence of obesity or being overweight and low-level physical activity. Substantial medical research points towards sugar-laden food and drinks as the culprit in the unprecedented increase of obesity cases, and in turn, in the prevalence of Type 2 diabetes. Ironically, cutting back on sugar intake only results in a small though significant effect on body weight.

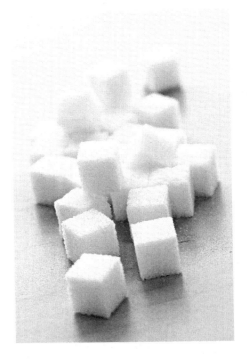

Some diabetics are probably sugar addicts, but even non-diabetics may also be suffering from sugar addiction. Sugar overload is toxic to the human body (see Chapter 3). Like any other toxins, it is imperative that excess sugar in the body be eliminated. This is the rationale behind this book on sugar detoxification (or detox) and this is explained further in Chapter 4.

How do you know if you need to undergo sugar detox? Chapter 1 provides you with the preliminaries and self-assessment questionnaires to evaluate whether or not you are suffering from sugar addiction and what type of sugar addiction you may be experiencing. There are four types of sugar addiction and the details are provided in Chapter 2. Meanwhile, Chapter 3 offers a primer on sugar detox, and Chapter 6 explains how even people who are not suffering from sugar addiction benefit from sugar detox.

Chapter 5 shows why sugar is dangerous for weight loss. A glimpse of natural alternatives for sugar is given in Chapter 7. Meanwhile Chapters 8, 9, and 10 comprise the core of the sugar detox method, with a special chapter on the significance of dermal detox in eliminating sugar toxins out of the body. Chapter 11 explains the connection between sugar and exercise. The maintenance plan to rid the body of sugar toxins after the detox plan is drawn in Chapter 12.

Tips on how to survive the detox process when you need to dine out are laid out in Chapter 13 because we know how dull life can be without a night out. Some yummy recipes are provided in the final chapter. Here's hoping for your successful detox. In no time, you will be healed of sugar addiction the natural way and your normal body functions will be restored. Enjoy reading and stay healthy and fit, folks!

Chapter 1: Preliminaries and Self-Assessment

The fine usually white, sweet crystals we call sugar appear harmless. After all, sugar comes from plants. Practically all plants make sugar for their own food aided by the process called photosynthesis. Sugar per se is, indeed, harmless. In fact, sugar plays important roles in the human body. However, the aforementioned statement should be properly qualified in terms of the type of sugar and the aspect of moderation.

Types of Sugar

Five types of sugar are described in sufficient this section: sucrose, fructose, glucose, lactose, and galactose. The other sugars will be enumerated. However, discussion will be limited to their classification as simple sugar or monossacharide, dissacharide, trisaccharides, etc. It is also important to remember that sugars are carbohydrates.

Sucrose

Table sugar, the form of sugar available in the market for consumers, is sucrose. The molecular formula of sucrose is $C_{12}H_{22}O_{11}$. It is a disaccharide, which is a combination of two simple sugars glucose and fructose. Sucrose is manufactured from sugar cane and sugar beets. More than two-thirds of manufactured today is from sugar cane.

The human body needs sucrose for energy. However, in terms of physical characteristics, not all sucrose is white crystals. There are 10 forms of commercially available sucrose:

- Baker's sugar: more finely granulated than fruit sugar;

- Brown sugar: sugar with molasses added;
- Confectioners' or powdered sugar
- Fruit sugar: very finely granulated sucrose (note is different from fructose which is commonly called fruit sugar, but is actually fruit and vegetable sugar);
- Invert sugar: very fine powdered sugar;
- Liquid sugar, a solution containing highly purified sugar and is used in canned foods and beverages;
- Muscovado or Barbados sugar, which is a finer brown sugar.
- Sanding sugar, which is a large granule sugar;
- Turbinado (amber colored) and demerara, which have slightly larger crystals and sometimes erroneously labeled as raw sugar; and
- White sugar, which is either fine or ultrafine (superfine), the most common sucrose used in the household.

Fructose

Fructose refers to natural sugar from fruits and vegetables. It is a simple sugar. People who consume a lot of fruits and vegetables in their diet have fructose as a major carbohydrate. The molecular formula of fructose is $C_6H_{12}O_6$, which is the same as glucose, another type of sugar. However, fructose and glucose are structurally different.

Fructose has three main functions in the body. Like sucrose, fructose also contributes to energy production. Another role of fructose is in the production of glycogen, which is responsible for the storage of carbohydrates for later use. Fructose also plays a role in fat storage for the body's future or emergency energy requirements.

Glucose

Glucose is also a simple sugar. It also constitutes an energy source. It is considered as the most significant sugar in the metabolism of humans. The recent discovery that glucose dangle from many body proteins and fats triggers significant positive and negative consequences. One of the most important new uses of glucose is in the development of treatment.

Lactose

Lactose is derived from milk and is alternately called milk sugar. It is a dissacharide consisting of the two simple sugars galactose and glucose. Its molecular formula is the same as sucrose ($C_{12}H_{22}O_{11}$). Lactose promotes the metabolism of fat, proteins, and minerals such as calcium, magnesium, and manganese.

Galactose

Galactose is a simple sugar (i.e., monossacharide) usually sourced in by the human body from the double sugar (i.e., disaccharide) lactose. It shares the same transport mechanism as glucose. Many of the structural elements of the human cells and tissues contain galactose.

Other Sugars

Sugars are structurally carbohydrates containing, carbon, hydrogen, and oxygen atoms. Other than the five kinds of sugar discussed above, which are either simple or double sugars (monossacharide or disaccharides), there are also polysaccharides such as starch from plants and animals, pectin, and cellulose, etc.

Moderation

Each person is a unique creation and, therefore has different dietary and nutritional requirements. What is moderate intake for one may be excessive for another or deficient for others. Moderation is therefore not only a frequently used phrased but also often misused, misinterpreted, and/or misunderstood. Moderation is the key to good health. However, moderation does not, in any way, preclude anyone from making necessary changes in their diet when they believe that they are eating in moderation.

Anything in this universe, sugar included, has a good side and a bad side. In fact, excessive drinking or eating of anything for that matter is bad for anyone. As far as sugar intake is concerned, some people may already be suffering from sugar addiction and they are not even aware of it. The mere fact that you are reading this book suggests that you are concerned about your sugar intake or you suspect that someone else, a family member or a loved one, may have problems related to sugar. The next sections presents a number of quizzes which may help you gain some information if you or someone you care about has sugar addiction.

Sugar Addiction Quizzes

Sugar addiction may be classified into four types. You may self-administer these quizzes or have someone you suspect to be a "sugar addict", take these exams. Knowing the type of sugar addiction one has can substantially aid in planning interventions. Remember, whatever the result of these quizzes, always have it checked by a medical practitioner specializing as a diabetologist or endocrinologist. However, the intervention being espoused in this eBook is safe as long as the instructions are correctly followed.

For all the four self-assessment quizzes, score yourself or someone you are evaluating for sugar addiction as 0 if the condition is not experienced. Otherwise, give the full score as indicated or instructed if the condition is experienced.

Quiz 1: Assessment for Type 1 Sugar Addiction

Put a check for each of the conditions you experience in the space provided for. After the quiz add up all your scores for the checked items and use the interpretation guide below the quiz labeled

"What your total score means" to find out if you have a problem with Type 1 sugar addiction.

	Do you experience the following conditions?	Score	Check Here
1.	I need coffee to get me going when I wake up every morning.	10	____
2.	I usually feel weak or experience low energy during the middle of the afternoon.	10	____
3.	I often suffer from indigestion.	15	____
4.	I have aches and pains here and there.	15	____
5.	I often suffer from headaches.	15	____
6.	I am almost always tired.	20	____
7.	I experience insomnia occasionally.	20	____
8.	I crave for sweets or coffee (or other drinks with caffeine) so that I will have energy for my daily routine.	25	____
9.	I gained weight and/or I am having difficulty losing the weight I gained during the past three years (Score this item equal to the number of pound you gained in 3 years. For example, if you gained 10 pounds in 3 years, this item will have a score of 10.).	____	____
10.	I drink ____ ounces of non-diet soda or non-decaf coffee everyday (Score this item equal to 2 times the number of ounces you indicated in the blank. For example, if you drink 12 ounces	____	____

each day, multiply 12 by 2 and write down 24 as your score.).

11. I work more than 40 hours per week. (Score this item equal to 2 times the number of hours you work more 40 hours. For example, if you work 48 hours per week, you have 8 hours in excess of 40. Multiply 8 by 2 and write down 16 as your score.). ____ ____

12. I drink ____ ounces of energy drinks containing sugar and/or caffeine everyday (Score this item equal to 6 times the number of ounces you indicated in the blank. For example, if you drink 8 ounces each day, multiply 8 by 6 and write down 48 as your score.). ____ ____

Add up the scores of all the items you checked: ____

What your total score means:

Total Score Range	Interpretation
0 to 40	Congratulations! You can relax for now. Your answers in Quiz 1 suggest that you do not have anything to worry about Type 1 sugar addiction. However, you are not done yet with the quizzes. Please take a deep breath and do some stretching before taking Quiz 2.
41 to 70	You have a problem with energy production, but the good news is: you are not sugar addicted. There are interventions to help you in this regard. Please read on.
71 and over	Your score indicates that you are somewhat

	dependent on sugar and caffeine for your energy production. Please read on. There are natural ways of restoring efficient energy production without charging your system with sugar and caffeine.

Quiz 2: Assessment for Type 2 Sugar Addiction

Put a check for each of the conditions you experience in the space provided for. After the quiz add up all your scores for the checked items and use the interpretation guide below the quiz labeled "What your total score means" to find out if you have a problem with Type 2 sugar addiction.

	Do you experience the following conditions?	Score	Check Here
1.	I experience sore throat and tend to have swollen glands every so often.	10	___
2.	I usually feel thirsty and had to urinate quite more frequently.	10	___
3.	I feel a substantial decrease in my energy level whenever I am stressed.	15	___
4.	I sometimes feel dizzy when I stand up.	15	___
5.	I feel that life is a crisis.	15	___
6.	I like the rush of energy when I am caught up in a crisis.	15	___
7.	I suffer from frequent and severe exhaustion, chronic fatigue syndrome or fibromyalgia when I have acute infection or whenever I am extremely stressed out.	25	___
8.	I practically turn into a hulk when I am hungry (in other words, I am extremely irritable when I feel hungry)	35	___

Add up the scores of all the items you checked: _____

What your total score means:

Total Score Range	Interpretation
0 to 24	You have healthy adrenal glands but your energy level is somewhat low-key or restrained.
25 to 49	Be careful. It looks like you are developing adrenal fatigue.
50 to 75	You need to get help if you have not done it yet. It is very likely that you are experiencing moderate adrenal exhaustion.
76 and over	You do not feel good about your health anymore and chances are, you feel terrible. Your symptoms suggest that you are either on your way towards severe adrenal exhaustion or you may already be suffering from it.

Quiz 3: Assessment for Type 3 Sugar Addiction

Put a check for each of the conditions you experience in the space provided for. After the quiz add up all your scores for the checked items and use the interpretation guide below the quiz labeled "What your total score means" to find out if you have a problem with Type 3 sugar addiction.

Do you experience (or did you experience) any of the following conditions?	Score	Check Here

1.	I am pregnant now (or I experienced pregnancy in the past).	5	____
2.	I had at least one course of antibiotics.	6	____
3.	I used to take birth control pills.	10	____
4.	I experience wheezing, teary or burning sensation in the eyes or any form of adverse reaction to the smell of perfume and other strongly-scented liquids or chemicals like insecticides.	10	____
5.	I experience the above symptoms more severely when I am exposed to damp or humid environment or when I am exposed to places infested with molds.	10	____
6.	I took corticosteroids such as Prednisone for more than one a month.	15	____
7.	I had fungal infection such as athlete's foot, jock itch, nail or skin infection which was difficult to treat?	20	____
8.	I took antibiotics for infection for over two consecutive months or short courses more than three times in a year.	20	____
9.	I have postnasal drip or I find it necessary to clear my throat a lot.	20	____
10.	I crave for sugar, bread or other forms of carbohydrates.	20	____
11.	I experience food allergies.	20	____
12.	I had prostatitis or chronic yeast vaginitis.	25	____

13. I have chronic fatigue syndrome or fibromyalgia.   50   ____

14. I have chronic nasal congestion or sinusitis.   50   ____

15. I experience spastic colon or irritable bowel syndrome (the symptoms are bloating, constipation and/or diarrhea, and gas).   50   ____

16. I experienced a condition (acne, for example) that needs to be treated with erythromycin, tetracycline or other antibiotics for a period of at least one month.   50   ____

Add up the scores of all the items you checked: ____

What your total score means:

Total Score Range	Interpretation
0 to 69	No clear symptoms of Type 3 sugar addiction. Conditions which generally lead to Type 3 sugar addiction were not reported.
70 or over	Conditions which generally lead to Type 3 sugar addiction are present. The assessment shows the possibility of a yeast/candida overgrowth.

Quiz 4: Assessment for Type 4 Sugar Addiction

For the last self-assessment quiz on sugar addiction, the checklist is different for each gender. Put a check for each of the conditions you experience in the space provided for. After the quiz add up all your scores for the checked items and use the interpretation guide below the quiz labeled "What your total score means" to find out if you have a problem with Type 4 sugar addiction.

For Women Only

| | Do you experience the following conditions related to pre-menstrual syndrome (PMS)? | Score | Check Here |

1. I experience either higher level or more severe symptoms such as anxiety, depression or unhappiness, bloating, and/or irritability one week or several days before my menstrual period (Score this item equal to 15 times the number of symptoms you experience. For example, if you have anxiety experienced severe irritability during the week before your period, multiply 2 by 15 and write down 30 as your score.). ____ ____

2. I have a history of PMS. 30 ____

Add up the scores of all the items you checked: ____

| | Do you experience the following conditions related to menopause or perimenopause? | Score | Check Here |

3. I observed a decrease in my libido or sex drive. 15

4. I experience either higher level or more severe symptoms such as fatigue, headache, hot flashes or profuse sweating, and/or insomnia one week or several days before my menstrual period or I generally

experience the aforementioned symptoms even if I no longer have my monthly periods. (Score this item equal to 20 times the number of symptoms you experience. For example, if you have experience insomnia and fatigue, multiply 2 by 20 and write down 40 as your score.).

5. I have reduced vaginal lubrication.   25   ____

6. I had hysterectomy or surgery involving my ovaries.   25   ____

Add up the scores of the last four items you checked: ____

What your total score means:

Total Score Range	Interpretation
PMS-Related Assessment	Your sugar cravings may be hormonal and if your score is 30 or higher, the information on possible interventions against sugar addiction can work wonders for your PMS. Kindly read on.
Assessment for Conditions Associated with Menopause or Perimenopause	Your sugar cravings may be hormonal and have something to do with changes related to menopause. If your score is 30 or higher, you are experiencing symptoms of either estrogen or progesterone deficiency. The information on possible interventions against sugar addiction can work wonders for your PMS. Kindly read on.

For Men Only: Only men 46 years or over generally experience symptoms for Type 4 sugar addiction. Younger males need not take this part of the sugar addiction assessment.

	Do you experience the following conditions related to pre-menstrual syndrome (PMS)?	Score	Check Here
1.	I have diabetes.	20	____
2.	I experience reduced ability to have erections or I have been diagnosed of erectile dysfunction.	20	____
3.	I have high cholesterol levels.	20	____
4.	I am suffering from hypertension.	20	____
5.	I experience reduced libido or sex drive.	20	____
6.	I am having fits of depression or having difficulty motivation myself in general.	20	____
7.	I am overweight or obese and I have a large belly or significantly increased waist measurement.	20	____

Add up the scores of all the items you checked: ____

What your total score means:

Total Score Range	Interpretation
0 to 39	No clear symptoms of Type 4 sugar addiction. Conditions which generally lead to Type 4 sugar addiction were not reported.

| 70 or over | Conditions which generally lead to Type 4 sugar addiction are present. The assessment shows the possibility of testosterone inadequacy. Kindly read on for possible safe interventions. |

Chapter 2 Sugar Addiction

An addiction is generally described as anything that a person must have in order to avoid a negative feeling or symptom. It may also be used to mean a compulsive tendency to produce or create a pleasurable sensation. Anyone can develop an addiction for just about anything and everything, even for objects which are otherwise harmless when consumed or used in moderation.

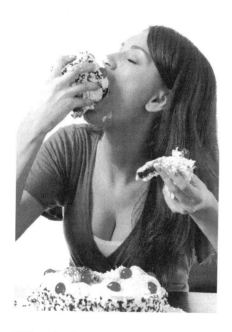

What is Sugar Addiction?

Sugar addiction is a condition where a person uses sugar to boost his/her energy to do away with the feeling of exhaustion or fatigue. People who turn to sugar as a mood lifter on a regular basis are also suffering from sugar addiction. As discussed in Chapter 1, sugar is mainly responsible for energy production. Sugar addicts depend on sugar to charge their system.

Likewise, sugar addicts also consume sugar to feel good because sugar triggers serotonin and dopamine production. These two hormones are responsible for feeling happiness and satisfaction. As with any other form of addiction, constant use of sugar to increase ones level of energy or to lighten up ones mood or feeling results in developing tolerance for it. Sugar adducts, therefore, need more and more sugar to experience the same rewards (i.e., feeling energetic and happy).

Types of Sugar Addiction

Sugar addiction is classified into four types based on their symptoms and general characteristics:

- Type 1 sugar addiction describes a condition where a person craves for sugar and caffeine to combat their chronic fatigue;
- Type 2 sugar addiction depicts a condition where a person is severely stressed in life and uses sugar to pump up his adrenal glands and help him/her handle the stressor;
- Type 3 sugar addiction illustrates a compulsion for sugar fixes several times a day because of an overgrowth of the toxic yeast Candida albicans; and
- Type 4 sugar addiction refers to the uncontrollable urge to consume high-sugar foods as a response to hormonal changes in the body.

Type 1
Type 1 sugar addicts have the penchant for perfection in whatever they do. Their drive for perfection takes its toll on their energy that is why they often have chronic fatigue. To succeed in their endeavors, they need an endless supply of energy to make things happen. Thus, they are usually hooked on coffee, sugar- and caffeine-laden energy drinks and sodas. However, the energy derived from the aforementioned drinks does not last long and usually makes people who consume them even more exhausted.

Moreover, sugar and caffeine is a troublesome team and causes a host of health problems. Among the adverse effects of high sugar and caffeine intake are chronic fatigue syndrome, fibromyalgia, headache, hypertension, impaired immune system, and sleeping disorders.

Type 2

Type 2 sugar addicts constantly react to environmental stressors. The body's natural stress relievers are activated in stressful situation - cortisol and adrenaline or epinephrine, which are produced by the adrenal glands. The adrenals, however, are not immune to all the stress it has to cope within a person's lifetime. Sometimes, it fails to provide that rush of energy people need to make them feel they are in control of the situation. Sugar addicts turn to sugar so that needed energy boost.

However, the surge of energy is short-lived and this is usually followed by a drop in the person's blood sugar. Glucose level in the blood drops which signals the brain that this person is hungry. If you remember the Incredible Hulk and the famous line: "Please don't make me angry; you wouldn't like me when I'm angry", you can change angry to "hungry" and you've got the Incredible Type 2 Sugar Addict. Nervous, anxious, jittery, irritable, and light-headed, the hulk needs to eat something sweet or all hells will break loose.

Type 3

Type 3 sugar addicts crave sugar from sunrise to sunset. This is because the undesirable yeast Candida albicans used the person's digestive system as a fermentation tank. The overgrowth of this yeast is even fed more by sugar intake. This heightens a sugar addict's craving for sweets into an uncontrolled fancy.

Type 4

Finally, Type 4 sugar addicts are depressed and like a tropical depression, they tend to crave for all the carbohydrates they lay their eyes on. This category of sugar addiction is not a consequence of stress, fatigue or yeast, but of changes in the level of sexual hormones. In the case of women who are at their worse during the week preceding their menstrual period or as they reach the period of menopause, the uncontrollable desire for sugar is a result of insufficient estrogen and progesterone. Meanwhile, in the case of men, those who are in their andropause period also tend to crave for sugar and have a substantial increase in their waistline. The condition is a result of insufficient levels of the male hormone testosterone.

There is Hope for the Sugar Addicts

The good news is, there is a proven and effective intervention for healing sugar addiction. The regimen consists of sugar detoxification (detox for short), exercise, hormones, immunity, nutrition, and sleep. The next chapter introduces the readers to the wonders of sugar detox.

Chapter 3 Sugar Detox

Sugar changes the composition of the mineral content of the blood. It particularly affects calcium, potassium, and sodium. Thus, the general consensus among health experts that refined sugar (i.e. table sugar) is one of the worse ingredients that humans take in is justified. Like other abused substances, the chemical reaction of refined sugar in the body acts as a poison and has a drug-lie effect. Sugar has many deleterious effects in the body and can cause a major imbalance in the body's organ systems. For this reason alone, people in general, and not just sugar addicts need to undergo sugar detoxification or sugar detox.

Like alcoholics and drug addicts, people suffering from sugar addiction should be rehabilitated. Sugar detox is rehabilitation from the harmful consequences of consuming too much sugar in the diet. It is, therefore, a good thing that the fundamentals of sugar detox is diet related. This does not suggest in any way that sugar detox will not pose difficulties to sugar addicts or even for healthy people who wish to experience the vaunted health benefits from sugar detox for that matter. In fact, using the so-called "cold turkey" approach to sugar addiction found success elusive without nutritional strategies.

What Is Sugar Detox?

The term detox is used interchangeably with cleanse to indicate a dietary plan that reduces or eliminates the consumption of unhealthy substances. Sugar detox is the process of cleansing the body of the harmful effects of sugar overload. Some of the harmful benefits of consuming sugar-loaded foods include:

- Sugar throws off the homeostatic imbalance of the whole body by increasing adrenaline production many times the normal capacity of the glands.

- It induces the nervous system to adopt the so-called "flight-or-fight" response which increases the production of cortisone, one of the two natural stress-busters of the body. Cortisone suppresses the body's immune function and this leads other health conditions.
- Sugar overload gives a person a false sense of energy. The feeling wears off after a short time and sugar addiction results from the body craving for sweets to have that energetic feeling. Increasing the body's sugar intake is a person's natural response when the body has developed tolerance for sugar. To get the fake energy rush, sugar addicts increase their consumption of sugar-laden foods more and more, until the cravings can no longer be controlled without nutritional/dietary intervention.

An Overview of Sugar Detox

Sugar, caffeine and flour comprise an unhealthy triune. Therefore, sugar detox usually incorporates methods to cleanse the body of caffeine and flour, too. For an effective sugar detox plan, one should also cut back on caffeine intake to at least half. Employ the "cold turkey" approach to sugar and flour. This involves totally eliminating these two ingredients in your diet. The best time to go on a sugar detox is NOW.

However, before deciding to do the detox plan, make sure you have the firm resolve to do it. If you cheat on your sugar and/or flour intake while on detox, your cravings will get more intense. By experience, sugar addicts who cheat fail in their detox goals.

Other important but basic components of the sugar detox plan include:

- Proteins such as eggs, protein shakes or butter from nuts, or nuts and seeds for breakfast.

- The healthy triune in sugar detox namely good carbohydrates, good fats, and good proteins. Examples of good carbs are fruit, beans and other vegetables, and whole grain foods. Meanwhile examples of good fats are avocadoes, extra virgin olive oil (authentic, there are a lot of fake ones in the market), fish, nuts, olives, and seeds. Eggs, fish, lean poultry, legumes, nuts, soy foods, and whole grains are good proteins.
- Small amounts of food taken more than thrice a day. Snacking helps you from feeling the fangs of hunger and starting a food binge. You may eat light every three hours. Almond, pumpkin or walnut seeds may be eaten raw or roasted dry (i.e., no oil or water).
- Eight glasses of clean and filtered water.

Chapter 4 Why Sugar Detox

There are a myriad of benefits which can be gained from sugar detox. These benefits are good for those suffering from sugar addiction and great for normal, healthy individuals as well. While candies, soda drinks, and irresistible pastries may not be toxic, per se, the same thing cannot be said of their refined sugar ingredient. It is not the intention of this eBook to scare you this much, but refined sugars and artificial sweeteners tend to impose a huge load of physiological stress on the body's systems. Believe it or not except for smoking, nothing matches the long term damage of sugar on the body.

A preview of the undesirable health consequences of sugar overload in the body was provided in Chapter 3. The details of the sneak preview are presented here together with the justification on the importance of sugar detox. The rationale for sugar detox includes medical or therapeutic benefits, as well as gains in terms of emotional, physical, and mental health.

In the first place, cleansing the body of sugar, which is also tagged as an "inflammatory devil" provides one with a jumpstart towards the path to weight loss, enhanced energy, more efficient immunity system, and superior nutrition. Detox also paves the way to quell one's cravings for sweets, enhance focus and improves mental clarity. With all the benefits of detoxifying the body of sugar, people will be well on their way to a more empowered and fulfilled life.

Medical or Therapeutic Benefits

Among the medical or therapeutic effects of sugar detox are: achieving normal blood sugar level and insulin control; prevention of post insulin sugar crash which causes fatigue and brain fog; restores normal thyroid and adrenal function; restores the body's intestinal flora to a healthy state to stimulate the production of immune cells and help metabolize dietary carcinogen; reduces inflammation and lowers the risk of diseases; and reduces bloating and gas.

Even if the body's inflammatory response is a necessary part of its physiology to heal wounds, fight infection, and rebuild the muscles. However, too much inflammation leads to a number of conditions such as Alzheimer's disease, atherosclerosis, arthritis, autonomous disorders, cancer, chronic pain, eczema, premature aging, and yeast infection. Sugar is an inflammatory food and having too much sugar in the body exposes it to a continuously inflamed state. Sugar detox helps prevent the foretasted conditions which put sugar addicts at a higher risk of contracting these conditions.

Physical Benefits

The physical benefits which can be derived from sugar detox include: higher energy level when detox is combined with mental exercise; maintenance of a vibrant lifestyle; prevention of diseases and illnesses; and better nutrition level towards good health.

Emotional and Mental Benefits

Sugar detox helps in reducing sugar cravings until the cravings are totally eliminated. The body's vitality will not depend anymore on a false sense of energy. When normal sugar level is reached or maintained one enjoys higher energy without caffeine or sugar overload.

Chapter 5 Why Sugar is Dangerous for Weight Loss

It will not be surprising at all if people with diabetes, particularly those who suffer from consistently above normal blood glucose levels to be diabetic and is struggling with their weight-loss regimen. Likewise, people with normal blood sugar levels may also be targeting an ideal weight range and are struggling with it. For both types off people who are into weight-loss plans, sugar poses grave danger.

Taking out sugar from your diet means that many high-calorie foods will have to be eliminated from your alternative menu. This results in a low carbohydrate diet. However, especially for diabetic patients, a low-carb diet is dangerous because of the risk of ketosis. Ketosis results when the body burns fat instead of carbs. So what is wrong with this, you may ask?

To achieve weight loss, sugar intake need to be restricted to as low as it is possible that will not endanger one's health. Many diets are anchored on maintaining the body in a ketogenic state to aid weight loss. However, this is not an all-encompassing principle. The glycemic index of foods which are to be included in a weight-loss diet plan should be considered. Moreover, the effect of the foods in the weight-loss menu should also take metabolic behaviors of low-glycemic foods.

When one is on a weight loss plan, food with low glycemic index is recommended. This is because food with high glycemic index tends to affect the glucose level of the blood (blood sugar) way more than foods with low-glycemic index (GI). Refined sugar has a GI of 60 and is classified under the medium GI sugars. Meanwhile, fructose has a significantly lower GI range between 12 and 23 or an average of less than 20.

High GI foods tend to result in blood sugar level fluctuations which cause more sugar cravings. More sugar cravings suggest more temptation to slip away from the diet and fail in the weight loss target goal. The danger of sugars for weight loss is not, however, confined to more sugar cravings.

Since fructose or fruit sugar has a low GI index, it is often extracted and manufactured as a white powder and labeled as natural low-GI sugar in the market. While fructose has low GI, it requires a special enzyme in the liver to metabolize it. This leaves the liver overworked. It is difficult for an overworked liver to achieve a state of ketosis for it to play its role in weight loss.

Chapter 6 Who will Benefit from Sugar Detox?

Sugar detox is for everyone. As discussed in the benefits of sugar detox, ridding the body of the deleterious effects of sugar is a concern for everyone. Particularly, detoxing from sugar provides a powerful head start towards shedding off unwanted weight and fat.

However, there is a special group of people who urgently need sugar detox for their conditions. This group includes:

- Individuals suffering from all four types of sugar addiction;
- Smokers who want to kick the habit;
- Those who are unsuccessful in kicking their sugar addiction using the cold turkey
- Diabetics;
- Patients suffering from hypertension
- Those who struggle with their excess weight;
- Individuals suffering from obesity;
- Those who dream of losing their spare tire on their abdomen (i.e., belly fat);
- People suffering from chronic fatigue;
- People whose unhealthy condition is brought about by chronic inflammation: congestive heart failure, fibromyalgia, fibrosis, heart attack, kidney failure, lupus, pancreatitis, psoriasis, stroke, surgical complications, etc;
- Individuals suffering from the following conditions: Alzheimer's disease, atherosclerosis, arthritis, autonomous disorders, cancer, chronic pain, eczema, premature aging, and yeast infection.

Chapter 7 Natural Sugar Alternatives

With the rampant and staggering statistics of diabetes cases sweeping every country in the world, pharmaceutical companies came to the rescue with artificial sweeteners. After all, what is life without sugar? However, it did not take very long for science to discover the dangers of long-term use of artificial sweeteners.

The Artificial Sweetener Scare: How They Work

Artificial sweeteners or synthetic chemicals that target the part of the brain that perceives the sweet taste of food or drinks. These chemicals work through the process of neuro-excitation. However, the active ingredient of these chemical tends to over-stimulate the brain neurons to the point that these neurons self-destruct. Thus, the chemicals in these artificial sweeteners commercially available widely cause damage to the users' brains. This adverse effect had been well-documented in research.

Artificial sweeteners works just like monosodium glutamate (MSG). It excites the brain's perception of taste to make people believe that food without MSG does not taste as good. MSG and artificial sweeteners were tagged as the primary cause of autism in children whose mothers were exposed to such chemicals.

The Best Natural Sweeteners

There are actually better alternatives to sugar than artificial sweeteners. Some of these safe natural sweeteners are discussed in this chapter. Among the top natural alternatives to sugar and artificial sweeteners are: stevia, xylitol, coconut palm sugar, and date sugar.

Stevia

Individuals who are suffering from diabetes, hypertension (high blood pressure), hypoglycemia, obesity or chronic yeast infection can benefit from stevia as sweetener without the usual drawbacks from artificial sweeteners. Stevia may be used to prepare your favorite sweets without having to welcome additional calories and without adversely affecting pancreatic and adrenal functions like sugar does. Moreover, it can satisfy sugar or carb cravings without having to worry about elevating blood glucose levels and putting on extra weight.

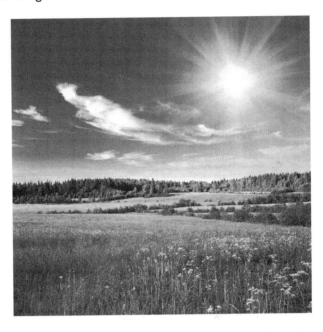

Stevia plantation: People can use manufactured stevia natural sweeteners or cultivate stevia in their garden for their own use.

Stevia is safe from children. Parents can even create sweet treats for their children using stevia to avoid childhood obesity, tooth decay and hyperactivity. For people accustomed to the taste of refined sugar, stevia may not be fair very well in comparison because of its licorice-like and somewhat transient bitter flavor. However, current technology can help improve the taste to eliminate the slight bitterness. Children should be trained at the earliest possible time with the taste of stevia to ensure that they don't get included in diabetes statistics.

Xylitol

You are probably familiar with xylitol because it has been successfully used as a natural sweetener for sugar-free chewing gum and candies. The good news is that xylitol is an all-natural substance which we produce in our own system during normal glucose metabolism. It can also be sourced from nature through berries, corncobs, lettuce, mushrooms, and hardwoods. Xylitol takes like sugar but with lesser calorie content and carbs. Moreover, teaspoon for teaspoon, it behaves like sugar when used in recipes. The only exception in its sugary characteristics is that it will not caramelize.

Xylitol does not increase the blood sugar level when ingested. It has a very low glycemic index at 7. It prevents tooth decay and the formation of plaque. It also promotes salivary flow to prevent damage to the tooth enamel. Xylitol also prevents osteoporosis and the development of streptococcus bacteria in the mouth and intestines.

Coconut Palm Sugar

This natural substitute to refined sugar is processed from the sap of the coconut palm tree. Coconut palm sugar is a mild sweetener but with low GI. It has a light caramel color. This sugar alternative dissolves just like brown sugar but lacks the strong flavor of molasses. Because of its low GI, it has less impact on the blood's glucose level that ordinary table sugar.

Date Sugar

This natural substitute to refined sugar is manufactured from ground dried dates. Besides its utility as a sweetener, it contains copper, iron, magnesium, and vitamins. Date sugar has that distinct date flavor which makes them delicious sugar substitutes in bread, cake, and muffins.

Chapter 8 The Sugar Detox Plan in a Nutshell: What to Eat, Not to Eat and How to Eat

Discussed here is the sugar detox plan. This chapter outlines what foods to eat and what not to eat. Also mentioned in a nutshell is the proper way of eating when in a detox plan. Moreover, some of the things which need to be done are also briefly discussed.

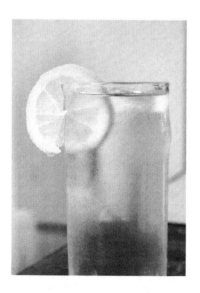

What to Eat and Drink

Water is basic to anybody-cleansing process. Drinking a minimum of 8 glasses (250 ml or approximately 8 ounces) of filtered or purified water is best for those to prefer an all-natural detox plan. However, those who are open to the idea of using a safe nutritional supplement, Cellfood may be added to drinking water so as to speed up the detox process. Put in 8 drops of Cellfood to one 250 ml water and do this three times each day, say two glasses of water with the supplement in the morning and another glass of water with the supplement before bedtime. The five or more glasses of water are taken without the supplement in between as desired.

The use of Cellfood in this eBook is not an endorsement of the supplement, but rather, an opinion based on this author's positive experiences in using it. It should be emphasized at this point that detoxing involves stirring up toxins stored in the body's stored part and other pertinent parts and organs of the body system. Using the oxygen supplement facilitates flushing out of the toxins and eliminating it. However, use of purified or filtered water is a "must". Otherwise, its full potency in the detox process will be reduced since it purifies water upon contact if the water has not been previously purified.

The benefits of using this nutritional supplement are three fold:

- It speeds up the process of detoxification, particularly in the blood lymphatic system and kidneys;
- It helps in the absorption of water by the cells; and
- It provides important nutrients, enzymes, and oxygen which are required for healthy detox.

Raw fruits and vegetables are essential in sugar detox. The enzymes, fiber, high quality protein, minerals, vitamins, and water content of fruits and vegetables will help provide the body' specific nutritional needs during the process. As much as possible, purchase organic fruits and vegetables. Otherwise, if you have no recourse but to have conventionally grown fruits and vegetables, these should be thoroughly washed. This is done to ensure that these crops will not expose you to more toxins from pesticides, bacteria, fungi, and mold.

The healthy triune in sugar detox namely good carbohydrates, good fats, and good proteins should be included. Examples of good carbs are fruit, beans and other vegetables, and whole grain foods. Meanwhile examples of good fats are avocadoes, extra virgin olive oil (authentic, there are a lot of fake ones in the market), fish, nuts, olives, and seeds. Eggs, fish, lean poultry, legumes, nuts, soy foods, and whole grains are good proteins.

The following foods are great for cleansing and should be eaten in controlled amounts or smaller than the normal servings:

- Apples
- Artichokes
- Avocadoes
- Bananas
- Beans
- Beets
- Blueberries
- Cabbage
- Carrots
- Celery and celery seeds
- Cherries
- Clarified butter
- Cranberries
- Eggs
- Fish
- Flaxseed and flaxseed oil
- Garlic
- Grapefruit
- Kale
- Legumes
- Lemons and limes
- Lentils
- Olive Oil
- Onions
- Organic free-range turkey
- Other seeds
- Quinoa
- Raspberries
- Sashimi
- Seaweed
- Tomatoes
- Wild caught salmon
- All other fruits and vegetables except potatoes

What to Not to Eat and Drink

Avoid meat as much as possible because is very acidic and requires tremendous energy to digest. However, if some people really have to eat some meat then the maximum meat intake is just a single serving in a week or two servings for the whole detox program of 1 day. A special condition for the small leeway on meat is that you should only purchase organic meat or poultry. Meat from cattle grown in the traditional method most probably contains toxins from the antibiotics and other medications as well as hormones which are fed to them to fatten them and keep them healthy.

Limit the intake of sweets to those prepared using natural sugar alternatives like stevia and xylitol only. Avoid synthetic sweeteners, including Nutrasweet or those using aspartame. The harmful effects of artificial sweeteners on the body make up a long list.

Never take alcohol and/or recreational drugs. Avoid smoking tobacco or cigarettes. Smokers who cannot help their cravings can benefit from the detox program in terms of reducing the cravings. Eventually, smokers can totally kick the habit.

Stay away from all foods and drinks with additives such as colors, flavor enhancers, preservatives, and stabilizers. Also avoid all wheat products. Even whole grains should be eating very sparingly.

Cut back coffee at least to half of your usual intake if you cannot do without it only for the first three days. After which, totally eliminate coffee from your diet. Also, avoid all soda, sweetened juices, fruit punch, and other sweetened or carbonated beverages.

The following foods should also be avoided:

- Agave nectar
- All fried foods
- Buckwheat
- Candy
- Cereal

- Cheese
- Cream sauces
- Dairy
- Evaporated canned juice
- Ezekiel bread
- Flour
- Flour tortillas
- Foods containing high-fructose corn syrup
- French bread
- Fructose
- Hydrogenated oils
- Maple syrup
- Millet
- MSG
- Oatmeal
- Potatoes
- Raw cane sugar
- Seitan
- Soy
- Sucrose
- Sugar
- Tortillas
- Trans fats
- Vinegar
- White rice
- Yogurt

Dos

Use prescription and over-the-counter drugs only when essential. Those who are on maintenance medication or are taking prescription drugs should consult with their doctors before attempting the detox process.

Exercise regularly but stay away from high-traffic or high-pollution area. This is necessary to prevent exposure to petrochemicals and other types of pollutants. Using a trampoline is good exercise for a detox program.

How to Eat

Small amounts of food should be taken more than thrice a day. Snacking helps you from feeling the fangs of hunger and starting a food binge. You may eat light every three hours. Almond, pumpkin or walnut seeds may be eaten raw or roasted dry (i.e., no oil or water).

Chapter 9 15-Day Meal Plan for Sugar Detox

Following is your 1-day meal plan for sugar detox. There are sample recipes in the last chapter (14). However, you can create your own sumptuous concoctions using Chapter 8 as guide. At least two more glasses of water should be taken within the day as desired by the person undergoing sugar detox.

DAY 1					
Breakfast	AM Snack	Lunch	PM Snack	Dinner	Late PM Snack
2 glasses water with supplement Fruit Vegetables Fish	1 glass water Fruit	1 glass water Cabbage and beans Mixed fruit desert (sugar free)	1 glass water Sugar-free desert	1 glass water with supplement 1 glass water Tomatoes and wild caught salmon	1 glass water Sugar-free desert
DAY 2					
Breakfast	AM Snack	Lunch	PM Snack	Dinner	Late PM Snack
2 glasses water with	1 glass water	1 glass water	1 glass water	1 glass water with	1 glass water

supplement Eggs	Walnut seeds	Carrot juice Organic free-range turkey	Quinoa	supplement 1 glass water Legumes Cranberries	Banana
DAY 3					
Breakfast	AM Snack	Lunch	PM Snack	Dinner	Late PM Snack
2 glasses water with supplement Sashimi Raspberries	1 glass water Flaxseeds	1 glass water Lemon juice Beets	1 glass water Cherries	1 glass water with supplement 1 glass water Legumes Cranberries	1 glass water Banana
DAY 4					
Breakfast	AM Snack	Lunch	PM Snack	Dinner	Late PM Snack

2 glasses water with supplement Sashimi Raspberries	1 glass water Flaxseeds	1 glass water Fruit Vegetables Organic poultry	1 glass water Almonds	1 glass water with supplement 1 glass water Kale Apple	1 glass water Grapefruit

DAY 5

Breakfast	AM Snack	Lunch	PM Snack	Dinner	Late PM Snack
2 glasses water with supplement Carrot cake using natural sweetener and clarified butter and coconut milk not	1 glass water Fruit or vegetable seeds not included in the "not to eat list"	1 glass water Fruit Vegetables Organic poultry	1 glass water Any fruit in season not included in that "not to eat list"	1 glass water with supplement 1 glass water Celery and other vegetables not included in that "not to eat list"	1 glass water Celery seeds

dairy Cherries				Banana		

DAY 6

Breakfast	AM Snack	Lunch	PM Snack	Dinner	Late PM Snack
2 glasses water with supplement Fruit in season not included in that "not to eat list" Mixed vegetables not included in that "not to eat list" Wild caught salmon	1 glass water Fruit or vegetable seed not included in that "not to eat list"	1 glass water Cabbage and carrots Banana	1 glass water Apple	1 glass water with supplement 1 glass water Tomatoes Salmon fish fillet (organics)	1 glass water Grapefruit

DAY 7

47

Breakfast	AM Snack	Lunch	PM Snack	Dinner	Late PM Snack
2 glasses water with supplement

Fruit in season not included in that "not to eat list"

Legumes and lentils

Steamed wild caught salmon | 1 glass water

Fruit or vegetable seed not included in that "not to eat list" | 1 glass water

Seaweed soup

Avocado | 1 glass water

Celery seeds | 1 glass water with supplement

1 glass water

Artichoke

Egg, onions, and garlic | 1 glass water

Quinoa |

DAY 8

Breakfast	AM Snack	Lunch	PM Snack	Dinner	Late PM Snack
2 glasses water with supplement	1 glass water

Flaxseeds | 1 glass water

Fruit

Vegetables | 1 glass water

Almonds | 1 glass water with supplement | 1 glass water

Grapefruit |

Sashimi Raspberries		Organic poultry		1 glass water Kale Apple	

DAY 9

Breakfast	AM Snack	Lunch	PM Snack	Dinner	Late PM Snack
2 glasses water with supplement Steamed carrots Turkey stew (organics)	1 glass water Walnut seeds	1 glass water Fruit Vegetables Organic poultry	1 glass water Banana	1 glass water with supplement Steamed cabbage and beans Egg omelet Blueberries	1 glass water Cherries

DAY 10

Breakfast	AM Snack	Lunch	PM Snack	Dinner	Late PM Snack
2 glasses water with suppleme	1 glass water Fruit or vegetab	1 glass water Fruit not included	1 glass water Any fruit in	1 glass water with suppleme	1 glass water Almonds

| nt
Carrot cake using natural sweetener and clarified butter and coconut milk not dairy

Cherries | le seeds not included in the "not to eat list" | in that "not to eat list"

Mixed vegetables not included in that "not to eat list"

Organic poultry in clarified butter | season not included in that "not to eat list" | nt
1 glass water

Legumes

Apples | |

DAY 11

Breakfast	AM Snack	Lunch	PM Snack	Dinner	Late PM Snack
2 glasses water with supplement Beets Sashimi	1 glass water Flaxseeds	1 glass water Fruit Vegetables Organic poultry	1 glass water Banana	1 glass water with supplement Steamed cabbage and beans Egg omelet	1 glass water Cherries

				Blueberries	

DAY 12

Breakfast	AM Snack	Lunch	PM Snack	Dinner	Late PM Snack
2 glasses water with supplement Fruit not included in that "not to eat list" Vegetables not included in that "not to eat list" Fish (organic)	1 glass water Fruit not included in that "not to eat list"	1 glass water Beans and organic poultry Mixed fruit desert (sugar free)	1 glass water Sugar-free desert	1 glass water with supplement 1 glass water Tomatoes and wild caught salmon	1 glass water Sugar-free desert

DAY 13

Breakfast	AM Snack	Lunch	PM Snack	Dinner	Late PM Snack
2 glasses water with	1 glass water	1 glass water	1 glass water	1 glass water with	1 glass water

supplement Fruit Vegetables Fish	Fruit	Cabbage and beans Mixed fruit desert (sugar free)	Sugar-free desert	supplement 1 glass water Tomatoes and salmon (organic) fillet	Avocado

DAY 14

Breakfast	AM Snack	Lunch	PM Snack	Dinner	Late PM Snack
2 glasses water with supplement Egg omelet Cranberries	1 glass water Pumpkin seeds	1 glass water Seaweed soup Organic fish	1 glass water Quinoa	1 glass water with supplement 1 glass water Lentils in olive oil Flaxseed	1 glass water Blueberries

DAY 15

Breakfast	AM Snack	Lunch	PM Snack	Dinner	Late PM Snack
2 glasses	1 glass	1 glass	1 glass	1 glass	1 glass

water with supplement Sashimi and seaweed Apples	water Flaxseeds	water Kale and legumes Apple	water Banana	water with supplement 1 glass water Lentils and cabbage Avocado	water Celery seeds

Chapter 10 Dermal Detox

You must be wondering why you are reading a chapter on dermal detox on a book about sugar detox. Firstly, this chapter is a necessary part of any detox program. God, indeed, has created a truly marvelous body for human beings. Under normal conditions, the body has its own detoxification process. However, unhealthy eating and lifestyle sometimes compromise the body's natural processes to rid itself of toxins. Be that as it may, the body still responds to human-initiated interventions to boost detoxification.

Channels of Detoxification

In the previous chapters, it was mentioned in passing that the liver and the kidney are channels of detoxification. They are, in fact, just two of the major pathways of detoxification. The other major pathways are the intestines and the lungs. Moreover, there are supporting channels of detoxification: the gall bladder, the lymphatic system, the blood, and the dermal system (i.e., the skin).

The skin is considered a secondary organ of detoxification or elimination. It is the largest of the elimination organs. The skin may be structurally considered as an organ because it is made up of tissues which are joined together to perform specific activities such as:

- Maintenance of body temperature
- Protection of the body from bacterial invasion, dehydration, and toxins and ultraviolet rays;
- Perception of stimuli;
- Excretion of wastes, salt, and organic compounds
- Synthesis of Vitamin D; and
- Bolstering of immunity.

The Skin's Role in the Detox Process

The skin aids in the body's natural detox process either by eliminating toxins from the inside or reacting with those from the outside so that once they enter the system, they would have already been neutralized or rendered inactive. Grounded on its large surface area, the skin is able to expel substantial amounts of cellular waste by eliminating them through the sweat glands and mucus secretions. In fact, the condition of the skin reflects the condition of everything beneath it.

The skin carries a larger-than-normal portion of waste for elimination in cases when the liver and the intestines are already overloaded. The skin is able to do this by throwing waste out of the body in the form of abscesses, acne, boils, pimples or rashes. During the sugar detox process, it is possible that skin eruptions such as the aforementioned conditions will appear. Do not be alarmed because those often unsightly eruptions are a sign that the detox process is in progress. In other words, it is a clear signal that the body is getting rid of toxins through its support channel of detoxification.

As the skin supports the detox process, you should also care and provide support to the skin by drinking enough purified water and better with added oxygen supplement. During the detox process, the skin will function well as a channel of elimination when it is brushed dry every day. There are also certain foods which facilitate dermal detox and enhance the skin condition.

To care for the skin, dry brushing using a natural bristle is recommended. Use a vegetable fiber brush instead of synthetic brush since the latter will scratch the skin. Dry brushing does not require the use of water. This helps the skin in eliminating toxins and opening pores through the shedding off of dead skin cells and removing other wastes. Brushing should be carried out in the morning as follows:

- Start at the bottom of your feet and move upward using circular motion until your reach your chest.
- Brush the abdomen using circular counterclockwise strokes.
- Move outward and inward starting with the hands going up the arms.
- Brush very lightly on your breasts and do not brush the nipples.
- For best results, brush the entire body.
- Use sea salt on the brush to help open the pores.
- Wash the brush every week and let it dry.

Dry skin brushing is not recommended for those suffering for skin conditions such as psoriasis and eczema. Saunas and steam baths are also helpful in releasing toxins through sweat. Therapeutics baths are also great for dermal detox. Use comfortably hot water and add specific ingredients such as Epsom salts, ginger, or baking soda with salt. Thalassotherapy or bathing in sea water is both therapeutic and detoxifying. Likewise, hot mineral springs are excellent for detox and relaxation.

The following foods help in the dermal detox process:

- Celery facilitates detox and blood circulation and promotes dermal flexibility;
- Cucumber enhances dermal elasticity;
- Lettuce helps restore damaged skin.

Chapter 11 The Sugar-Exercise Connection

To maintain a state of ketosis, avoid products with a high glycemic index as well as products that are metabolized primarily by the liver. Strawberries and blueberries are naturally high in fructose and may not help sustain a ketogenic diet. However, fructose is found in varying degrees in all fruits, vegetables and many processed foods. Although it cannot be avoided altogether, incorporating physical activity into your daily routine may help provide some allowance for certain fruits given that you work your body hard enough to deplete the glycogen storage in the muscle.

Recommended Exercise for Sugar Detox

Aerobic exercise is great not only for sugar detox but also for dermal detox. Among the recommended dermal exercises are:

- Fast walking, which enhances circulation and enhance perspiration to promote the excretion of toxins through the skin more efficiently; and
- Use of home video exercise workouts, especially those that incorporate the use of hand weights, is an excellent way to get started with exercise, if exercise is not a regular thing in your daily routine.

Benefits of Exercise in Sugar Detox

Exercise is a staple in the natural detox process. It boosts metabolism and elevates body temperature. An increase in temperature promotes vasodilatation, which in turn, regulates blood circulation. Exercise also aids in balancing the body's blood pH level for a more health alkalinic blood. Exercise also oxygenates the body cells to enhance the immune system.

The Sugar-Exercise Connection

A healthy immune system is especially important in sugar detox since it is the immune system that combats yeast infection. Exercise also helps lower the blood glucose levels to help fight against yeast infection. This is one aspect of the sugar-exercise connection.

Moreover, exercise facilitates removal of toxins from the deleterious effects of sugar overload. Additionally, the effect of exercise on the lymphatic system promotes elimination of toxins from the cell. Regular exercise helps the pathways of detoxification in filtering out the toxins. A good metabolism ensures that the liver, kidneys and other organs are not overworked so that they will be effective in the detox process. This is the second link in the sugar-exercise connection.

Chapter 12 Maintenance Plan

It is not a bad thing to go on with the detox diet for more than 15 days. However, if you are raring to have some leeway on the foods to avoid, having a glucose monitor is necessary. Constantly monitoring your GI will help you observe which particular foods are significantly affecting the increase. That is, if eating a little serving of foods to avoid raises your blood sugar level. However, you cannot take in sugar right after the detox plan.

Monitoring your blood sugar while experimenting on certain foods on the avoid list will give you a fairly good idea if it is OK for you to eat some of these foods sparingly. If your GI increases even after taking the readings 2 to 3 hours after the meal, avoid that food. If you need to eat meat, purchase organic-grown cattle and poultry. Additionally, you need to exercise regular to help your body use up any extra sugars that you are ingesting. If your blood sugar is constantly 25% higher than your blood sugar than after the detox program. Go on another round of detox.

Chapter 13 How to Dine Out with Sugar Detox Diet

Being on a detox diet does not necessarily mean that you need to totally shun dining out. Socialization with friends and family is vital to your emotional health. Normally you would not initiate an invitation to dine out while on detox. However, your friends may invite you for one or more dine-outs in a week while you are on detox. Don't worry.

You do not have to say no for dine-outs every so often. This is true most especially if you intend to go on periodic detox diets regularly. Here are some tips on how to dine out even when on a sugar detox diet:

Research beforehand about what options are available on the designated restaurants by calling them before the dine-out date. If it's a consolation, there are restos which have gluten-free food in their menu. Among these restaurants are: Diverso by Ferraro, Il Fornello, Magic Oven, and Pizza Pizza.

If there is no specific restaurant on the dine-out invitation, you may suggest a restaurant that has available option for people who are on a diet plan.

- For restaurants which allow options for clients on diet, just perform some basic calculations and substitutions to get the healthy salad allowed for your detox diet plan.
- Vegetarian restos are usually the best options for people who are on specific diets. Schedule your dine-outs in this type of restaurants.
- You may suggest a house party instead use your garden or another friend's garden for the party. The party may even be a potluck, and you can contribute a meal on the menu prepared in accordance with your detox plan. You can even

spice up the fun by distributing guidelines pertaining to food and ingredients to bring on the potluck. Who knows, your friends may even be interested to undergo the sugar detox plan themselves.
- Finally, cheating with a nibble in your friend's chosen restaurant will not hurt that bad. Just drink more water, and sweat it out through exercise. Chapter 14

Chapter 14 Some Sugar Detox Recipes

Tomato Relish

Ingredients:

- 4 tomatoes
- 1 lime
- 1 mild green chili
- 1 red onion
- a handful of mint
- a pinch of salt
- a dash of finely ground black pepper

Procedure:

Cut the tomatoes in 4 pieces, take out the seeds and chop finely.

Juice the lime.

Chop the red onion finely.

Deseed and chop the green chili finely.

Finely chop the mint

Put all the ingredients in a bowl and stir until well combined.

Spicy Fruit Mix

Ingredients:

- 1 large apple (juiced)
- 1 large bell pepper (juiced)
- 2 cups frozen strawberries or any other berries in the "what to eat list"
- 1 lemon juiced
- a pinch of cayenne

Procedure:

Blend all the ingredients until smooth. Serves 2

Fruit and Veggie Mix 1

Ingredients:

- 1 cup carrot juice
- 2 frozen bananas
- 1 cup walnut milk
- 1 teaspoon cinnamon
- 1 teaspoon vanilla extract
- a pinch of sea salt

Procedure:

Blend all the ingredients until smooth. Serves 2

Zesty Fruit Mix

Ingredients:

- 1 banana
- 2 cups fresh or frozen blueberries
- 1-1/2 cups nut milk of choice
- 2 probiotic capsules (to boost digestion and metabolism)

Procedure

Blend all the ingredients until smooth. Serves 1 to 2

Made in the USA
Lexington, KY
25 October 2018